UNBREAKABLE POWER OF THE BRAIN

A Guide to Optimizing Your Brainpower, Enhance Your Memory, Focus, and Creativity

Charles Porras

Copyright

All rights reserved. No part of this publication may be reproduced, distributed, or transmitted in any form or by any means, including photocopying, recording, or other electronic or mechanical methods, without the prior written permission of the publisher, except in the case of brief quotations embodied in critical reviews and certain other noncommercial uses permitted by copyright law.

Copyright © Charles Porras, 2024.

Disclaimer

The information contained in this book is intended for educational purposes only and is not a substitute for medical advice, diagnosis, or treatment. Please consult with a qualified healthcare professional regarding any questions or concerns you may have about your brain health or any condition you may be experiencing.

The authors/editors/contributors of this book make no guarantees or warranties with respect to the accuracy, completeness, or applicability of the content presented. The use of the information in this book is at your own risk.

Gratitude page

Dear Reader,

Thank you for choosing **"Unbreakable power of the brain"**! We're absolutely delighted to welcome you on this incredible exploration of the universe within. The human brain is a fascinating and complex organ, and we're confident this journey will be both enlightening and empowering.

Inside **this book,** you'll discover the latest scientific insights into how your brain works, from the formation of memories to the spark of creativity. We'll delve into the power of neuroplasticity, your brain's remarkable ability to change and adapt throughout life.

But **"Unbreakable power of the brain"** isn't just about theory. We'll equip you with practical strategies to optimize your brain health and unlock its full potential. You'll learn how to:
- Enhance your memory and focus with powerful techniques.
- Boost your cognitive function through simple lifestyle changes.
- Cultivate creativity and critical thinking skills.
- Manage stress and protect your brain from its negative effects.
- Embrace lifelong learning and keep your mind sharp for years to come.

We believe that everyone deserves to understand and harness the incredible power of their brain.

This book is your guide to a healthier, happier, and more fulfilling life.

With gratitude,
Charles Porras.

Table of contents

Introduction **6**
   The Brain 7
   The Power of Change: concept of neuroplasticity 9

Chapter 1 .... **12**
The Mastermind and Its Minions **12**
   Analyzing the brain's structure 12
   A symphony of parts 14

Chapter 2 .... **18**
The Orchestra of the Mind **18**
   Breakdown of the brain's major functions 18
   From sight to perception 21
   Fun fact files 23

Chapter 3 .... **26**
The Memory Maze **26**
   Types, formation and retrieval of memory 26
   Why can't I remember where I parked my car?.. 29
   Boosting your memory palace 31

Chapter 4 .... **34**
The Power of Focus **34**
   Attention, please! 34
   Taming the inner chatterbox 37
   Sharpening your mental focus 41

Chapter 5 .... **46**
The Emotional Rollercoaster **46**
   The amygdala and the limbic system 46
   Why do emotions feel so powerful? 49

Language of emotions...................................... 52
　　　Managing your emotional landscape.............. 54
Chapter 6... 58
When the Brain Goes Awry................................ 58
　　　Mental health matters..58
　　　Neurological disorders................................... 61
　　　The impact of brain injuries............................64
Chapter 7... 68
Fueling Your Brain Machine................................68
　　　The brain on a diet... 68
　　　Move it or lose it!.. 71
Chapter 8... 73
Keeping Your Brain Sharp.................................. 74
　　　Lifelong learning...74
　　　Brain-training games and activities................ 77
　　　Sleep for success...82
Chapter 9... 86
Taming Stress and Embracing Mindfulness.... 86
　　　The stress monster and the brain.................. 86
　　　Relaxation techniques for a calmer you..........89
Chapter 10... 92
The Cutting Edge of Brain Research................. 92
　　　Exploring the frontiers..................................... 92
　　　Ethical considerations..................................... 95
Conclusion.. 96

Introduction

Derek was a happy and active child until a terrible car accident at the age of 7 left him with a traumatic brain injury (TBI). Doctors told his family the damage was extensive, affecting movement, speech, and cognitive abilities. They believed his recovery would be very limited.

Derek's parents, however, refused to give up. They enrolled him in intensive therapy programs, focusing on physical rehabilitation, speech therapy, and cognitive exercises. The process was grueling, filled with frustration and setbacks. Yet, Derek persevered, fueled by an unwavering determination to regain his independence.

The power of his brain was remarkable. Despite the damage, it began to form new connections and rewire itself. Slowly, Derek started regaining some movement in his limbs. He relearned how to speak, word by painstaking word. His cognitive abilities, while not entirely back to normal, showed significant improvement.

Years later, Derek's story is one of triumph. He walks with a cane, speaks clearly, and even graduated from high school with honors. He may not have full use of his body, but his brain's resilience has allowed him to live a full and meaningful life. He is a motivational speaker, inspiring others facing challenges and showcasing the unbreakable potential of the human brain.

Derek's story exemplifies the book's theme perfectly. Even after a severe injury, the brain has the astonishing ability to heal, adapt, and find new ways to function. It's a testament to the human spirit's will to overcome adversity and the remarkable power of the brain to defy limitations.

The Brain

Have you ever stopped to think about the most powerful computer you own? It's not your laptop or smartphone – it's nestled right inside your skull, weighing about three pounds, and wrinkled like a forgotten walnut. This seemingly unassuming blob of tissue, the brain, is the most complex organ in the human body, and it's the very foundation of who you are.

Imagine a bustling metropolis, a city that never sleeps. Billions of tiny citizens, called neurons, constantly fire electrical messages back and forth across a trillion intricate pathways. This symphony of activity is the brain in action, coordinating everything from the simplest muscle movement to the most profound philosophical thought.

The brain's complexity is truly mind-boggling. It holds onto every memory you've ever made, from the taste of your grandmother's cookies to the lyrics of your favorite childhood song. It regulates your emotions, making you laugh until your sides ache or cry until your heart feels heavy. It allows you to learn new skills, solve problems, and create art that moves others.

In short, the brain is the control center of your existence. It shapes your personality, your desires, and your very perception of the world. It's the reason you can dream up fantastical stories, solve complex equations, or feel a surge of love when you see a loved one's face.

But despite its incredible power, the brain remains a bit of a mystery. We're still unlocking its secrets, understanding how these billions of neurons work together to create the magic of consciousness. This book is an invitation to embark on a journey of discovery, to delve into the fascinating world of the brain and explore its unbreakable power.

The Power of Change: concept of neuroplasticity

For decades, the prevailing belief was that the brain, like a meticulously sculpted statue, was fixed and unchanging after childhood. But a revolutionary concept is shattering this misconception: **neuroplasticity**. This term refers to the brain's remarkable ability to adapt, rewire itself, and form new connections throughout life.

Imagine the brain not as a rigid structure, but as a dynamic landscape. With experience and learning, new pathways are forged between neurons, like trails carved by persistent hikers. Conversely, unused pathways fade away, just like untrodden paths become overgrown. This constant rewiring allows the brain to constantly learn, adapt, and even heal from injury.

Think about a child learning to ride a bike. At first, it's a wobbly, dangerous process. But with practice, the brain forms new connections between the motor cortex, cerebellum, and sensory areas, resulting in smooth, effortless riding. This is neuroplasticity in action!

Here's the truly empowering part: neuroplasticity isn't limited to childhood. It's a lifelong process. An adult learning a new language, a senior citizen taking up painting, or even someone recovering from a stroke – all are examples of the brain's incredible ability to adapt and improve, even later in life.

Neuroplasticity challenges the notion of a fixed intelligence or an unchangeable personality. It empowers us to believe that with dedication and effort, we can continuously learn, grow, and unlock new potentials within our brains. This concept forms the core principle of this book. We'll explore how to harness the power of neuroplasticity and unlock the brain's unbreakable potential for change and growth at any stage of life.

Unbreakable power of the brain

Chapter 1
The Mastermind and Its Minions

Analyzing the brain's structure

Imagine a three-pound control center nestled within your skull, intricately folded and wrinkled like a well-worn map. This is your brain, the most complex organ in the human body, and it's about to be demystified! Let's embark on a journey to understand the key players in this remarkable structure:

The Cerebrum

- This is the largest part of the brain, accounting for about two-thirds of its weight. It's like the CEO, overseeing all higher-level functions.
- Divided into two hemispheres, left and right, each with specialized skills:
    - **Left hemisphere:** Think of the left hemisphere as your analytical powerhouse. It's the maestro of language, allowing you to understand and produce speech, read, and write. It

       also excels in mathematical calculations and logical reasoning, helping you solve problems and make decisions based on facts.
    o **Right hemisphere:** The right hemisphere is your creative counterpart. It's where imagination takes flight, processing visual information, music, and emotions. It plays a crucial role in spatial awareness, helping you navigate your surroundings and understand complex visual patterns.

- The cerebrum is further divided into lobes, each with specific responsibilities. We'll explore these lobes in more detail later.

The Cerebellum

- While smaller than the cerebrum, the cerebellum is no less important. Nicknamed the "little brain," it's responsible for coordinating your movements, maintaining balance, and ensuring smooth muscle control. It's the reason you can walk without wobbling, catch a ball with ease, and maintain perfect posture.

The Brainstem

- Located at the base of the brain, connecting it to the spinal cord, this is the mission control for our most basic functions.
- It regulates essential activities like breathing, heart rate, digestion, and even sleep-wake cycles. Without the brainstem, life wouldn't be possible.

By understanding these key regions and their functions, we gain a foundational appreciation for the intricate machinery that keeps us functioning.

A symphony of parts

Imagine an orchestra. Each instrument plays its own unique role, but together they create a harmonious symphony. The brain functions in a similar way. While we've identified distinct regions like the cerebrum, cerebellum, and brainstem, their true power lies in their **collaborative effort**. Let's look into how these different parts work together to produce complex behaviors:

- **The Cerebral Cortex:** Think of the cerebral cortex, particularly the frontal lobe, as the conductor of the brain's orchestra. It receives information from various regions, analyzes it, and initiates commands. It's responsible for planning, decision-making, and integrating information from different sensory areas.
- **The Sensory Ensemble:** Our senses – sight, sound, touch, taste, and smell – constantly bombard the brain with information. Specialized areas in the cortex, like the visual cortex or the auditory cortex, process this sensory data. Imagine the visual cortex as the section that translates the light hitting your retina into a clear image you see.
- **The Relay Racers:** The information processed by the sensory areas doesn't stop there. It's relayed through a network of pathways called white matter to other brain regions for further analysis and integration. These pathways act like relay racers, carrying the baton of information from one region to another.
- **The Emotional Orchestra Pit:** The limbic system, nestled deep within the brain, plays a crucial role in processing emotions. It interprets the sensory information received and triggers our emotional responses. For example, when you see a delicious cake, the visual cortex sends signals to the limbic system, triggering feelings of pleasure and desire.
- **Putting Thoughts into Action:** Finally, the translated and integrated information reaches the

motor cortex, located in the back of the frontal lobe. This area is the brain's command center for movement. It sends signals to your muscles, allowing you to react and move purposefully – like reaching out to grab that delicious slice of cake.

This collaborative effort is what allows us to experience the world in a rich and meaningful way. Imagine seeing a beautiful sunset. The visual cortex processes the colors and shapes, while the limbic system evokes feelings of awe and wonder. Meanwhile, the frontal lobe might prompt you to capture the scene on camera, sending signals to your motor cortex to coordinate your movements.

Unbreakable power of the brain

Chapter 2
The Orchestra of the Mind

Breakdown of the brain's major functions

The human brain is a magnificent orchestra, a complex network of billions of neurons working in perfect harmony to produce the symphony of our existence. Each region plays a vital role, contributing to the incredible range of functions that make us who we are. Let's delve deeper into the brain's major functions and understand how they work together to create this masterpiece:

1. Cognition

The frontal lobe, particularly the prefrontal cortex, acts as the maestro of the brain's orchestra. It's responsible for our higher-order cognitive functions, including:

- **Planning and Decision-Making:** The prefrontal cortex analyzes information, weighs options, and formulates plans for action. It allows us to think strategically, solve problems, and make well-informed choices.

- **Memory:** Different brain regions contribute to memory formation, retrieval, and consolidation. The hippocampus plays a crucial role in forming new memories, while the frontal lobe is involved in working memory, allowing us to hold information in our minds for short periods.
- **Learning:** The brain is constantly learning and adapting. When we encounter new experiences, our neurons form new connections, strengthening our understanding of the world. The hippocampus and prefrontal cortex are key players in this process.
- **Language:** Language processing is a complex feat. Broca's area is responsible for speech production, while Wernicke's area helps us understand spoken language.

2. Motor Skills

The motor cortex, located in the back of the frontal lobe, is responsible for initiating and coordinating our movements. It sends signals to our muscles, allowing us to perform everything from simple tasks like walking to complex actions like playing a musical instrument. The cerebellum also plays a crucial role in fine-tuning our movements and maintaining balance.

3. Sensory Processing

Our senses – sight, sound, touch, taste, and smell – constantly bombard the brain with information.

Specialized areas in the brain process this sensory data, creating our perception of the world:

- **Vision:** The occipital lobe is the primary visual processing center. It receives signals from the retina and translates them into the images we see.
- **Audition:** The temporal lobe is responsible for processing sound. It allows us to distinguish different pitches, volumes, and recognize familiar sounds like music or speech.
- **Touch, Taste, and Smell:** The somatosensory cortex processes information about touch, pressure, and temperature. The gustatory cortex and olfactory cortex handle taste and smell, respectively.

4. Emotional Regulation

Deep within the brain lies the limbic system, a group of structures responsible for processing emotions. It interprets the sensory information we receive and triggers our emotional responses. The amygdala plays a key role in processing fear and aggression, while the hippocampus helps us consolidate emotional memories. The prefrontal cortex also plays a role in regulating our emotions and helping us respond appropriately.

5. Autonomic Functions

The brainstem and hypothalamus work tirelessly behind the scenes, controlling our autonomic functions – the involuntary processes that keep us alive.

These include regulating our heart rate, breathing, digestion, sleep-wake cycles, and even body temperature.

From sight to perception

Close your eyes for a moment. Imagine a juicy, ripe strawberry. Can you almost taste its sweetness? This vivid experience, though conjured in your mind, is a testament to the brain's incredible ability to process sensory information and create our perception of the world.

Let's go deeper into this fascinating process, taking sight as an example:

1. Capturing the Light: Our journey begins with light reflecting off an object and entering our eyes. The light hits the retina, a light-sensitive layer at the back of the eyeball.

2. Transduction: Light into Signals: Specialized cells in the retina called photoreceptors (rods and cones) convert the light energy into electrical signals. These signals travel through the optic nerve to the brain.

3. The Thalamus: Relay Station The optic nerve relays the electrical signals to the thalamus, a sensory relay center in the brain. The thalamus acts like a switchboard, directing the signals to the appropriate processing area.

4. The Visual Cortex: Where Sight Takes Shape: The primary visual cortex, located in the occipital lobe, is the brain's headquarters for processing visual information. Here, the electrical signals are transformed into a meaningful representation of the visual world. Different areas within the visual cortex specialize in processing specific aspects of an image, such as color, shape, movement, and depth.

5. Beyond the Primary Cortex: Putting the Pieces Together: The visual information is further processed in higher-order visual areas. These areas integrate information from different parts of the visual cortex and from other sensory areas (like touch) to create a unified perception.

6. Perception: The Grand Illusion: Our perception of the world isn't just a passive reflection of sensory information. The brain actively interprets and constructs our reality based on past experiences, emotions, and expectations. This is why two people can look at the same strawberry and have slightly different perceptions of its color, size, or ripeness.

The Magic of Integration:

Creating a complete and unified perception of the world goes beyond just processing individual senses. The brain integrates information from all our senses to create a cohesive experience. For example, when you see a steaming cup of coffee, the visual cortex processes the image, while the olfactory cortex might conjure up the aroma of freshly brewed coffee. This multi-sensory integration allows us to have a richer and more meaningful experience of the world around us.

Fun fact files

Get ready to have your mind blown with these fascinating facts about the brain!

Fact File 1: A Shocking Misunderstanding!

For centuries, people believed the heart, not the brain, was the center of intelligence. Ancient Egyptians even removed the brains during mummification rituals, believing the heart held the key to a person's thoughts and memories! Thankfully, science eventually prevailed, and we now know the brain reigns supreme.

Fact File 2: Laughter – The Universal Language?

Laughter truly is the best medicine! But did you know it also activates both the left and right hemispheres of the brain? This might explain why humor is so contagious –

it triggers a synchronized response in the brains of those around us. So next time you share a laugh, you're not just creating a happy moment; you're engaging in a fascinating brain-to-brain connection!

Fact File 3: The Brain's Marathon – Running on Fumes (Almost)!

Our brains are incredibly energy-hungry organs, consuming a whopping 20% of the body's total energy, even though they only represent about 2% of our body weight! That's like a tiny computer using more power than a desktop! Thankfully, the brain primarily runs on glucose (sugar) from our bloodstream, ensuring it has the fuel it needs to function optimally.

Fact File 4: The Multitasking Myth!

While we might juggle multiple tasks throughout the day, our brains aren't actually multitasking. Instead, they're rapidly switching focus between different tasks, creating the illusion of multitasking. This constant context switching can actually decrease efficiency and increase the risk of errors. So, next time you have an important task, give your brain a break by focusing on one thing at a time.

Fact File 5: The Smell Connection – More Than Just Delicious!

Our sense of smell might not be as strong as some animals, but it still plays a crucial role in our lives beyond just detecting pleasant aromas. The olfactory bulb, located deep within the brain, has a direct connection to the limbic system, which processes emotions and memories. This explains why certain smells can evoke powerful emotional responses, transporting us back to a specific time and place in our lives. The next time you catch a whiff of freshly baked cookies and feel a wave of nostalgia, remember, it's your brain making the connection!

Chapter 3

The Memory Maze

Types, formation and retrieval of memory

Memories are the cornerstones of our identity. They shape who we are, influencing our decisions, emotions, and even our perception of the world. But how exactly do we form and retrieve these memories? The answer lies in the brain's remarkable memory system, a complex interplay of different types of memory and intricate processes. Let's embark on a journey to unveil this fascinating mystery:

The Players on the Memory Stage:

- **Short-Term Memory:** Imagine holding a phone number in your mind just long enough to dial it. That's the realm of short-term memory, a fleeting storage system that holds a limited amount of information for a brief period (usually seconds to minutes) without conscious effort.
- **Working Memory:** Think of working memory as your mental workspace. It allows you to hold

and manipulate information from short-term memory, like juggling multiple tasks or following complex instructions.
- **Long-Term Memory:** This is the holy grail of memory, the vast library within your brain that stores information for long periods, from childhood experiences to factual knowledge. Long-term memory can be further categorized into:
  - **Declarative Memory:** This is your conscious memory for facts and events. It can be further divided into episodic memory (specific events from your life) and semantic memory (general knowledge about the world).
  - **Non-declarative Memory:** This encompasses unconscious skills and habits, like riding a bike or playing a musical instrument.

The Memory Formation Process:

1. **Encoding:** This is where the magic begins. For information to be stored in long-term memory, it first needs to be encoded or processed into a form the brain can understand. This often involves paying attention, making connections to existing knowledge, and using strategies like rehearsal or mnemonics.
2. **Consolidation:** Once encoded, memories are fragile and susceptible to forgetting. Consolidation is the process of strengthening

these memory traces, making them more permanent. Sleep plays a crucial role in consolidation, allowing the brain to solidify newly formed memories.
3. **Storage:** Consolidated memories are then stored in various brain regions depending on the type of information. The hippocampus plays a central role in forming new memories, while other areas store specific types of information, like the visual cortex for visual memories.

The Art of Retrieval:

Remembering something is like pulling a book off a library shelf. Retrieval involves accessing the stored information and bringing it back to conscious awareness. Cues and prompts play a critical role in this process. For example, the smell of freshly baked cookies might trigger a childhood memory of baking with your grandma. The more elaborately a memory is encoded, the easier it is to retrieve later.

The Memory Maze: Why We Forget

Forgetting is a natural part of the memory process. Sometimes, retrieval cues are weak, or memories haven't been consolidated strongly enough. Interference from other memories can also make it difficult to recall specific information. The good news is that we can improve our memory by employing strategies that enhance encoding, retrieval, and overall brain health.

Why can't I remember where I parked my car?

We've all been there. You rush out of the store, bags overflowing, mind preoccupied with your grocery list. You reach the parking lot, a sinking feeling creeping in – you can't remember where you parked your car! This seemingly simple memory lapse is a fascinating example of how our memory system works, and sometimes doesn't.

Here's why your car might be playing hide-and-seek in the parking lot:

The Encoding Enigma:

Let's rewind to the moment you parked. Were you distracted by a phone call, a screaming child, or the internal debate between organic kale and regular lettuce? When we're not paying close attention, information isn't encoded effectively into short-term memory. This fragile stage is crucial for transferring information to long-term storage. Without proper encoding, your car's location becomes a blurry detail lost in the sea of recent events.

The Retrieval Roadblock:

Even if you encoded the parking spot somewhat, retrieval can be tricky. Imagine the parking lot as a massive library. You know the car is there (the memory is stored), but without a clear retrieval cue (remembering where you parked), finding it can be like searching for a specific book without a title or author.

The Interference Intersection:

Perhaps you parked next to a bright red car, similar to one you saw earlier that day. This creates "interference" – competing memories that can make it difficult to pinpoint the exact location of your own car.

The Memory Maze: Not a Sign of Forgetfulness

This parking lot predicament doesn't necessarily mean you have a bad memory. It simply highlights the complexities of our memory system. Here are some tips to avoid future car-finding fiascos:

- **Conscious Encoding:** Actively pay attention to where you park. Take a mental note of landmarks or your floor number in a multi-story parking lot.
- **Mnemonic Magic:** Use a memory trick like visualizing your car parked next to a specific store or a funny-looking car.
- **Repetition is Key:** Take a moment to review where you parked before leaving the store. This strengthens the memory trace and makes retrieval easier.

By understanding the different stages of memory and the factors that can influence them, we can develop strategies to improve our memory and avoid those frustrating "where-did-I-park?" moments. So, the next time you park your car, take a mindful moment to encode its location. Your future self (and your sanity) will thank you for it!

Boosting your memory palace

The human brain is a powerful memory machine, but sometimes it needs a helping hand. Luckily, there are a number of strategies you can employ to improve your memory recall, strengthen memory consolidation, and transform your memory palace into a place of effortless retrieval.

Strategies for Sharper Memory

- **Active Engagement:** Don't passively absorb information. Pay close attention, take notes, and ask questions. Engaging with the material strengthens the memory trace.
- **Make Connections:** Connect new information to existing knowledge. This creates a mental web, making it easier to remember and retrieve information later. Use mind maps, analogies, or personal anecdotes to create these connections.
- **Elaborate and Organize:** Don't just memorize facts in isolation. Take the time to elaborate on them, understand their significance, and

organize them in a logical way. This deeper processing strengthens the memory encoding.

Forging Lasting Memories

- **Sleep on It:** Sleep plays a crucial role in memory consolidation. Getting enough quality sleep allows the brain to solidify newly formed memories and transfer them to long-term storage. Aim for 7-8 hours of sleep each night.
- **Spaced Repetition:** Reviewing information at spaced intervals, rather than cramming right before a test, strengthens memory consolidation. Use flashcards or spaced repetition apps to revisit key concepts at increasing intervals.
- **Practice Retrieval:** Don't just passively reread information. Actively test yourself by recalling facts, summarizing concepts, or explaining them to someone else. This retrieval practice strengthens the memory and makes it more accessible in the future.

Advanced Techniques

- **Mnemonics Magic:** Use mnemonic devices like acronyms, rhymes, or peg words to encode information in a memorable way. For example, the acronym HOMES can help you remember the five Great Lakes (Huron, Ontario, Michigan, Erie, Superior).
- **Method of Loci Mastery:** This powerful memory technique involves associating

information with specific locations in a familiar place. Imagine your house and mentally place each item you need to remember in a specific room or location. When you need to recall the information, mentally walk through your house and "pick up" the items you placed there.
- **Visualization Power:** Engage your senses! Create vivid mental images, funny scenarios, or even outrageous stories to associate with the information you want to remember. The more bizarre or memorable the image, the easier it will be to recall later.

Remember, consistency is key! By incorporating these strategies into your daily routine, you can gradually improve your memory and unlock the full potential of your memory palace. With dedication and practice, you'll be well on your way to becoming a memory master!

Chapter 4

The Power of Focus

Attention, please!

Imagine a bustling city street. Cars honk, people chatter, and music spills from cafes. Somehow, you manage to focus on your friend's conversation amidst the sensory overload. This remarkable ability to filter incoming information and focus on specific aspects of our environment is thanks to our brain's attention system. Let's delve deeper into the science of attention and how it acts as a spotlight within our vast mental landscape.

The Attention Bottleneck:

Our brains are bombarded with sensory data every second. Sight, sound, touch, smell, and taste constantly send signals vying for our attention. However, our cognitive processing abilities are limited. This creates an "attention bottleneck" – the brain's inability to process all incoming information simultaneously. Here's how the brain filters and prioritizes:

- **Selection by Salience:** Certain things naturally grab our attention. Loud noises, bright lights, or

sudden movements activate brain regions that trigger a "fight-or-flight" response or signal something important in our environment.
- **Top-Down Control:** Our goals and expectations also play a crucial role. If you're looking for a specific book in a library, your attention will be drawn to books with relevant titles or colors, filtering out the rest.
- **Habituation:** Repeated stimuli tend to fade into the background. The constant hum of traffic eventually becomes less noticeable as your brain habituates to it. This allows you to focus on the conversation with your friend.

Types of Attention:

There are two main types of attention that work together:

- **Focused Attention:** This is the spotlight mode, where you concentrate on a specific task, like reading a book or solving a math problem. It requires effort and can be disrupted by distractions.
- **Divided Attention:** This is the ability to attend to multiple tasks simultaneously, like listening to a lecture while taking notes. However, divided attention often comes at a cost – performance on both tasks may suffer.

The Benefits of a Well-Trained Attention System:

A well-trained attention system is crucial for learning, memory, and overall cognitive function. It allows us to filter out distractions, focus on important tasks, and process information efficiently. However, attention can be susceptible to various factors:

- **Fatigue:** A tired brain struggles to focus, making us more susceptible to distractions.
- **Stress:** Chronic stress can impair attention and make it difficult to concentrate.
- **Technology:** The constant barrage of notifications and stimuli from our devices can fragment our attention and make it harder to focus on sustained tasks.

Sharpening Your Attentional Spotlight:

The good news is that we can train our attention system to function more effectively. Here are some tips:

- **Mindfulness Meditation:** Regular meditation practice can improve focus and reduce mind-wandering.
- **Minimize Distractions:** When tackling important tasks, silence your phone notifications, find a quiet space, and minimize clutter on your desk.
- **Schedule Breaks:** Our attention naturally wanes over time. Schedule short breaks to refresh your focus and come back to the task feeling recharged.
- **Prioritize Sleep:** Getting enough quality sleep is crucial for optimal brain function, including attention. Aim for 7-8 hours of sleep each night.

The Players on the Attention Stage:

- **The Thalamus:** This sensory relay center acts as a switchboard, directing incoming sensory information to different brain regions for processing.
- **The Reticular Activating System (RAS):** This network of neurons acts like a volume knob, regulating the level of alertness and filtering out irrelevant sensory information.
- **The Prefrontal Cortex:** This region, located behind the forehead, plays a crucial role in top-down processing, directing our attention based on goals, expectations, and past experiences.

Attention and Learning:

The ability to focus and direct our attention is crucial for learning. When we pay attention to information, it's processed more deeply and is more likely to be stored in long-term memory. Conversely, distractions can significantly hinder learning and memory formation.

Taming the inner chatterbox

Ever sit down to work, only to find yourself lost in a mental labyrinth of to-do lists, past conversations, or upcoming social events? This constant internal chatter can be a major roadblock to focus and productivity. But fear not, fellow warriors against distraction! This section looks into powerful techniques like mindfulness and meditation, equipping you to tame the inner chatterbox and achieve laser focus.

Mindfulness: The Art of Observing Your Thoughts

Mindfulness is the practice of paying attention to the present moment without judgment. It's like stepping back and observing the constant stream of thoughts and sensations that bombard your mind, rather than getting caught up in them. This simple act of awareness can be a powerful tool for managing distractions. Here's how:

- **Becoming Aware of the Chatter:** The first step is to simply become aware of the inner chatter. Notice the endless to-do lists, worries about the future, or judgments about the past that constantly swirl in your mind. Don't try to force these thoughts away, simply acknowledge them with a gentle curiosity.
- **Detachment from the Noise:** Once you've acknowledged the thoughts, practice detaching from them. Imagine them as leaves floating down a stream, observing them as they pass by without getting swept away in their current.

- **Anchoring Your Attention:** With practice, you can learn to gently guide your attention back to the present moment. This could be focusing on your breath, the sensations in your body, or the sounds around you. As you anchor your attention in the present, the inner chatter loses its power to distract you.

Meditation: Training Your Focus Muscle

Meditation is like a gym for your attention muscle. By regularly practicing meditation techniques, you can strengthen your ability to focus and resist distractions. There are many different meditation styles, but here's a simple one you can try:

- **Find a Quiet Space:** Sit comfortably in a quiet space where you won't be interrupted.
- **Set a Timer:** Start with a short meditation session, like 5 minutes, and gradually increase the duration as you become more comfortable.
- **Focus on Your Breath:** Close your eyes or soften your gaze. Bring your attention to your breath, feeling the rise and fall of your chest or abdomen with each inhalation and exhalation.
- **The Inevitable Wandering Mind:** It's natural for your mind to wander. When you notice yourself lost in thought, gently bring your attention back to your breath without judgment.
- **Observe and Return:** Meditation isn't about achieving a blank mind. It's about observing the

thoughts that arise and then gently returning your attention to your focus point (your breath).

Integrating Mindfulness and Meditation into Your Daily Life

The beauty of these techniques is that they can be practiced anywhere, anytime. Even a few minutes of mindful breathing throughout the day can significantly improve your focus and help you manage distractions. Here are some ways to integrate these practices:

- **Mindful Mornings:** Start your day with a short meditation session to set the tone for focus and clarity.
- **Mindful Breaks:** During your workday, take short mindfulness breaks to refocus and recharge. Simply close your eyes, take a few deep breaths, and observe your thoughts without judgment.
- **Mindful Tech Use:** Be mindful of how technology affects your focus. Schedule dedicated times to check emails and social media, and avoid distractions when tackling important tasks.

By incorporating mindfulness and meditation into your daily routine, you can quiet the inner chatterbox, sharpen your focus, and transform your mind into a laser beam of productivity.

Sharpening your mental focus

Feeling scatterbrained and easily distracted? You're not alone! The modern world bombards us with information and stimuli, making it challenging to maintain focus. But fear not! Here are some practical exercises and strategies you can employ to sharpen your mental focus and conquer distractions:

Exercise Your Focus Muscle:

- **The Pomodoro Technique:** This time management method involves working in focused 25-minute intervals with short breaks in between. Set a timer for 25 minutes, work on a single task with laser focus, then reward yourself with a 5-minute break. Repeat this cycle for several rounds. This technique trains your brain to maintain concentration for short bursts and helps prevent burnout.
- **The Two-Minute Rule:** For small tasks that are tempting distractions, apply the two-minute rule. If a task can be completed in two minutes or less, do it immediately rather than letting it linger on your mind. This helps clear your mental space and prevents small distractions from snowballing.
- **Mindfulness Games:** There are many online and mobile apps that offer brain-training games that can improve focus and attention span. These games often involve tasks like visual tracking, memory challenges, or rapid decision-making.

Tame the Technology Dragon:

- **Silence Notifications:** During focused work periods, silence notifications from emails, social media, and other apps. These constant pings and alerts fragment your attention and make it difficult to maintain focus.
- **Schedule Tech Breaks:** Don't let technology control your schedule. Schedule specific times to check emails and social media, instead of letting them interrupt your workflow.
- **Declutter Your Digital Workspace:** A cluttered desktop or disorganized files can be visually distracting. Organize your digital workspace, close unnecessary tabs, and create a clean environment that promotes focus.

Optimize Your Environment:

- **Minimize Clutter:** A cluttered physical workspace contributes to mental clutter. Tidy your desk, eliminate unnecessary distractions, and create a clean and organized environment conducive to focused work.
- **Natural Light is Your Friend:** Studies show natural light can improve focus and concentration. If possible, position your workspace near a window or consider using a light therapy lamp to mimic natural sunlight.
- **Optimize for Comfort:** Ensure your workspace is comfortable. Adjust your chair height, lighting, and temperature to create an

environment that minimizes physical discomfort and allows you to focus entirely on the task at hand.

Fuel Your Focus:

- **Hydration is Key:** Dehydration can negatively impact focus and cognitive function. Drink plenty of water throughout the day to stay hydrated and maintain optimal brain function.
- **Healthy Food Choices:** Just like your car needs the right fuel, your brain needs the right nutrients to perform at its best. Choose brain-boosting foods like fruits, vegetables, whole grains, and lean protein to fuel your focus.
- **Limit Sugar and Caffeine Crashes:** While a sugary snack or a strong cup of coffee might provide a temporary energy boost, the subsequent crash can significantly impair focus. Opt for sustained energy sources and avoid sugary treats or excessive caffeine.

Prioritize Sleep:

- **Aim for Quality Sleep:** A well-rested mind is a focused mind. Aim for 7-8 hours of quality sleep each night. Regular sleep allows your brain to consolidate memories, recharge, and prepare for optimal focus the following day.
- **Develop a Relaxing Bedtime Routine:** A consistent sleep schedule and a relaxing bedtime

routine help signal to your body that it's time to wind down. This promotes better sleep quality and ultimately enhances your focus the next day.

Unbreakable power of the brain

Chapter 5
The Emotional Rollercoaster

The amygdala and the limbic system

Our emotions aren't fleeting feelings; they are complex responses orchestrated by a network of brain regions known as the limbic system. At the heart of this emotional processing center lies the amygdala, a tiny but powerful structure that plays a crucial role in generating, regulating, and expressing emotions. Let's delve deeper into this fascinating collaboration:

The Limbic System:

Imagine the limbic system as an orchestra, with each region playing a specific instrument in the grand symphony of emotions. Here are some key players:

- **Amygdala:** The amygdala acts like the conductor, integrating sensory information, assessing potential threats, and triggering emotional responses. It's the first responder in emotional processing, responsible for generating feelings like fear, anger, and excitement.

- **Hippocampus:** This region plays a vital role in memory and learning. The amygdala can tag emotionally charged memories with a stronger emotional imprint, making them more likely to be remembered vividly.
- **Hypothalamus:** This structure acts as a bridge between the nervous system and the endocrine system. When the amygdala detects a threat, the hypothalamus triggers the fight-or-flight response, releasing hormones like adrenaline to prepare the body for action.
- **Cingulate Gyrus:** This region helps us become aware of our emotions and plays a role in emotional regulation.

The Amygdala: From Fear to Fury

The amygdala is particularly adept at processing emotions related to fear and survival. When faced with a potential threat, the amygdala triggers a rapid emotional response, preparing the body to react swiftly. This "amygdala hijack" can sometimes lead to impulsive reactions before we've had a chance to rationally assess the situation.

Regulating the Emotional Orchestra

Thankfully, the limbic system doesn't operate in isolation. The prefrontal cortex, the area responsible for higher-order thinking and reasoning, can act as a conductor for the amygdala. When we encounter a situation that triggers an emotional response, the prefrontal cortex can intervene, helping us to regulate our emotions and respond in a more measured way.

Understanding the Link Between Brain and Behavior

By understanding the interplay between the amygdala and the limbic system, we gain valuable insights into human behavior. This knowledge can be applied to various aspects of life, from managing stress and anxiety to developing emotional intelligence and building stronger relationships.

Here are some additional points to consider:

- **Individual Differences:** The amygdala's size and activity can vary between individuals, influencing their emotional reactivity and sensitivity.
- **The Impact of Experiences:** Early life experiences can shape the way the amygdala functions. For example, childhood trauma can lead to a heightened emotional response.

Why do emotions feel so powerful?

Emotions aren't just fleeting feelings; they're powerful motivators that color our thoughts, guide our actions, and leave a lasting imprint on our memories. But what makes them feel so intense? The answer lies in the intricate dance between the biological underpinnings of emotions and their influence on our cognitive processes.

The Biological Spark:

Our emotional experiences are orchestrated by a complex network of brain regions, with the amygdala taking center stage. This almond-shaped structure acts as an emotional alarm system, rapidly processing sensory information and triggering responses based on their perceived threat level. Here's the biological cascade that ignites our emotions:

1. **Sensory Input:** We encounter a situation (e.g., seeing a spider) or receive information (e.g., bad news) that triggers a sensory response.
2. **The Amygdala Takes Charge:** The amygdala receives this sensory information and, based on past experiences and evolutionary wiring, interprets it as a potential threat (fear of spiders) or a negative event (sadness from the bad news).
3. **Hormonal Response:** The amygdala communicates with the hypothalamus, which in turn activates the nervous system and endocrine system. This releases hormones like adrenaline (preparing you to fight or flee the spider) or

cortisol (the stress hormone associated with sadness).
4. **Physiological Changes:** These hormonal changes produce the physical sensations we associate with emotions. Your heart might race, your breathing quicken, or you might feel a surge of energy (fight-or-flight response).

Emotions Hijacking the Thinking Train:

The speed and intensity of this biological response is what makes emotions feel so powerful. They can hijack our rational thinking processes, often leading to impulsive reactions before the prefrontal cortex, the area responsible for higher-order thinking, has a chance to intervene. This explains why we might blurt out something hurtful in anger or freeze in fear when faced with a perceived threat.

The Emotional Influence on Cognition:

Emotions don't just affect our immediate actions; they also influence how we think and remember. Here's how:

- **Emotional Attention Filter:** Emotions act as a filter for incoming information. We tend to pay more attention to stimuli that are congruent with our current emotional state. Feeling happy? You might notice joyful faces in a crowd more readily. Feeling anxious? You might hyperfocus on potential dangers.
- **Emotional Memory Boost:** Emotionally charged memories are more vivid and

long-lasting. The amygdala can tag these memories with a stronger emotional imprint, making them easier to recall. This is why a traumatic experience from childhood might feel so real even after many years.
- **Emotional Decision-Making:** Emotions play a significant role in decision-making. Fear might lead us to avoid a situation, while excitement might push us to take risks.

Understanding the Power of Emotions:

By understanding the biological basis of emotions and their influence on our thoughts and actions, we can harness their power for good. Here's how:

- **Emotional Awareness:** Developing emotional intelligence allows us to recognize our emotions and understand their triggers.
- **Emotional Regulation:** Once we're aware of our emotions, we can develop strategies to manage them effectively. Relaxation techniques, mindfulness practices, and healthy coping mechanisms can help us respond thoughtfully instead of reacting impulsively.
- **Emotional Intelligence in Relationships:** Understanding emotions in ourselves and others fosters empathy and strengthens relationships.

Emotions are a fundamental part of the human experience. By appreciating their biological roots and their impact on our cognitive processes, we can navigate the world with greater self-awareness and emotional intelligence.

Language of emotions

Emotions are powerful, but they can also be complex to express and understand. Thankfully, language plays a crucial role in navigating this emotional landscape. But how does the brain translate the raw feeling into spoken or written words? Here, Broca's and Wernicke's areas, the powerhouses of language processing, come into play.

The Language Processing Duo:

- **Broca's Area:** Located in the left frontal lobe, Broca's area is primarily responsible for speech production. It plays a key role in formulating our thoughts into coherent sentences and selecting the appropriate words to express ourselves. When processing emotional language, Broca's area helps us articulate the feelings we experience.
- **Wernicke's Area:** Situated in the left temporal lobe, Wernicke's area is responsible for language comprehension. It allows us to understand the emotional language of others. When someone expresses their feelings verbally or in writing,

Wernicke's area helps us decipher the emotional content of their message.

The Emotional Connection:

While Broca's and Wernicke's areas are traditionally associated with general language processing, they also play a role in the specific domain of emotional language. Here's how:

- **Understanding Emotional Nuance:** Wernicke's area goes beyond just comprehending the literal meaning of words. It helps us pick up on subtle cues like tone of voice, facial expressions, and body language, which are all crucial for understanding the emotional undercurrent of communication.
- **Expressing Emotions Clearly:** Broca's area isn't just about stringing words together. It also helps us choose words that accurately convey the emotional intensity and nuance of our feelings. This allows us to express joy, sadness, anger, or any other emotion in a way that resonates with the listener.

Damage and Disruption:

Damage to Broca's or Wernicke's area can disrupt our ability to process emotional language. Here are some potential consequences:

- **Broca's Aphasia:** Individuals with damage to Broca's area might struggle to find the right words to express their emotions, even though they understand the feeling itself. They might use simpler language or have difficulty forming complex sentences to convey their emotional state.
- **Wernicke's Aphasia:** People with Wernicke's area damage might have difficulty understanding the emotional content of spoken or written language. They might misinterpret the emotional tone or miss subtle cues that convey feelings.

Managing your emotional landscape

Life throws emotional curveballs. From everyday frustrations to significant challenges, navigating the ups and downs can feel overwhelming. But fear not! We all have the potential to become skilled emotional landscape architects, cultivating resilience and fostering healthy emotional regulation. Here are some tips and techniques to empower you:

Emotional Regulation: Calming the Inner Storm

- **Mindfulness and Meditation:** Mindfulness practices like meditation can help you become aware of your emotions without judgment. By

observing your thoughts and feelings without getting caught up in them, you can gain a sense of control and respond thoughtfully instead of reacting impulsively.
- **Deep Breathing Exercises:** When emotions run high, deep breathing techniques can activate your body's relaxation response. Focus on slow, controlled breaths to calm your nervous system and bring your emotions back to a manageable level.
- **Identify Your Triggers:** Pay attention to situations, people, or events that tend to trigger strong negative emotions. Once you identify your triggers, you can develop coping mechanisms to navigate them effectively.
- **Positive Reframing:** Challenge negative thought patterns that fuel emotional turmoil. Try reframing situations in a more positive light or focusing on the aspects you can control.
- **Healthy Outlets:** Find healthy outlets for expressing your emotions. Talk to a trusted friend, therapist, or keep a journal to process your feelings in a constructive way.

Building Resilience: Strengthening Your Emotional Core

- **Building a Support System:** Surround yourself with positive and supportive people who uplift you and create a safe space for you to express your emotions.

- **Develop Healthy Habits:** Prioritize activities that nourish your mind and body. Regular exercise, a balanced diet, and quality sleep all contribute to emotional well-being and resilience.
- **Practice Gratitude:** Taking time to appreciate the good things in life, big or small, can shift your focus towards positivity and cultivate a sense of optimism, even in challenging times.
- **Learn from Setbacks:** View challenges as opportunities for growth. Reflect on what you learned from a difficult experience and use that knowledge to navigate future hurdles with greater resilience.
- **Self-Compassion is Key:** Treat yourself with kindness and understanding. Everyone experiences negative emotions; self-compassion allows you to navigate them without harsh self-criticism.

Remember, consistency is key! Building emotional regulation skills and resilience takes time and practice. By incorporating these techniques into your daily routine, you'll gradually develop the emotional intelligence and strength to navigate your emotional landscape with greater ease.

Here are some additional points to consider:

- **Seek professional help:** If you're struggling to manage your emotions or cope with difficult

situations, don't hesitate to seek professional help from a therapist or counselor.
- **Celebrate your progress:** Acknowledge and celebrate your progress, no matter how small. Every step towards emotional regulation and resilience is a victory!

By taking charge of your emotional landscape, you can cultivate a sense of inner peace, navigate challenges with greater strength, and build a more fulfilling and emotionally healthy life.

Chapter 6
When the Brain Goes Awry

Mental health matters

Mental health is an integral part of overall well-being. Just as physical illnesses can affect the body, mental health conditions can impact the brain's function and chemistry. Let's delve into how three common conditions – depression, anxiety, and schizophrenia – affect the brain:

Depression:

Depression is a mood disorder characterized by persistent feelings of sadness, loss of interest, and changes in appetite and sleep. Here's how it can affect the brain:

- **Reduced Neurotransmitters:** Depression is often linked to a decrease in certain neurotransmitters, like serotonin and norepinephrine, which play a crucial role in regulating mood, motivation, and pleasure.
- **Hippocampal Shrinkage:** The hippocampus, essential for memory and learning, can shrink in individuals with depression. This can lead to

difficulty concentrating, forming new memories, and feeling hopeful about the future.
- **Increased Activity in the Amygdala:** The amygdala, which processes emotions like fear and sadness, can become hyperactive in depression. This can contribute to feelings of negativity and hopelessness.

Anxiety:

Anxiety disorders are characterized by excessive worry, fear, and physical symptoms like rapid heart rate and shortness of breath. This is how anxiety affects the brain:

- **The Amygdala on High Alert:** Similar to depression, the amygdala plays a key role in anxiety. In anxious individuals, the amygdala is overly sensitive to perceived threats, triggering the fight-or-flight response even in non-threatening situations.
- **Imbalance in Neurotransmitters:** Anxiety can be linked to an imbalance in neurotransmitters like GABA, which has calming effects, and glutamate, which is excitatory. An imbalance can lead to difficulty relaxing and feeling overwhelmed.
- **The Prefrontal Cortex Takes a Backseat:** The prefrontal cortex, responsible for rational thinking and emotional regulation, can struggle to control the overactive amygdala in anxiety disorders. This can lead to difficulty controlling worries and calming down.

Schizophrenia:

Schizophrenia is a severe mental disorder characterized by hallucinations, delusions, and disorganized thinking. It affects brain function in several ways:

- **Dopamine Dysregulation:** Schizophrenia is often linked to abnormal activity in the dopamine system. Dopamine is a neurotransmitter involved in reward, motivation, and movement. Dysregulation can lead to hallucinations and difficulty filtering out irrelevant sensory information.
- **Reduced Gray Matter:** Individuals with schizophrenia may have reduced gray matter volume in certain brain regions, including those involved in perception, thought processing, and emotional regulation.
- **Connectivity Issues:** The brain's communication pathways between different regions may be disrupted in schizophrenia. This can contribute to difficulties with thinking, planning, and social interaction.

It's important to note:

- These are simplified explanations of complex brain processes.
- The exact causes of these conditions are not fully understood, and they likely involve a combination of genetic and environmental factors.

- There is no single brain abnormality that defines any of these conditions.
- Brain imaging can be a helpful tool for diagnosis, but it cannot definitively diagnose a mental health condition.

The good news?

The brain has remarkable plasticity, meaning it can change and adapt throughout life. With proper treatment, including medication, therapy, and lifestyle changes, people with these conditions can experience significant improvement and manage their symptoms effectively.

Neurological disorders

The nervous system, with the brain as its command center, controls everything from our thoughts and movements to our sensations and memories. When malfunctions occur in this intricate network, they can manifest as neurological disorders. Here, we'll explore three common conditions – dementia, Alzheimer's disease, and Parkinson's disease – to understand how they disrupt brain function:

Dementia: An Umbrella Term

Dementia is a broad term encompassing a decline in cognitive function that interferes with daily life. It's not a specific disease, but rather a collection of symptoms caused by various underlying conditions. Here's the key takeaway:

- **Symptoms:** Dementia can affect memory, thinking, reasoning, communication, and the ability to perform daily activities. The severity of symptoms varies depending on the underlying cause.

Alzheimer's Disease: The Memory Thief

Alzheimer's disease is a progressive neurodegenerative disorder, meaning brain cells deteriorate over time. It's the most common cause of dementia, a decline in cognitive function that significantly impacts daily life. Here's how it affects the brain:

- **Plaque and Tangles:** Hallmark features of Alzheimer's are the buildup of protein fragments called beta-amyloid plaques and tau tangles within brain cells. These disrupt communication between neurons and lead to cell death.
- **Hippocampal Atrophy:** The hippocampus, critical for memory formation and retrieval, shrinks significantly in Alzheimer's. This explains the progressive memory loss associated with the disease.

- **Neurotransmitter Decline:** Levels of acetylcholine, a neurotransmitter vital for memory and learning, decline in Alzheimer's brains. This contributes to cognitive decline and difficulty with tasks like remembering recent events or following conversations.

Parkinson's Disease: The Movement Thief

Parkinson's disease is another neurodegenerative disorder primarily affecting the part of the brain responsible for movement control. Symptoms include tremors, stiffness, and difficulty with balance and coordination. Here's how it disrupts the brain:

- **Loss of Dopamine Neurons:** In Parkinson's, dopamine-producing neurons in the substantia nigra region of the brain degenerate. Dopamine is crucial for initiating and coordinating movement.
- **Lewy Bodies:** These abnormal protein clumps accumulate in the brain cells of individuals with Parkinson's. They disrupt the function of remaining dopamine neurons and contribute to movement difficulties.
- **Secondary Effects:** As the disease progresses, other brain regions involved in mood, sleep, and thinking can also be affected. This can lead to depression, sleep disturbances, and cognitive decline in some patients.

Important Considerations:

- While dementia, Alzheimer's, and Parkinson's are common, there are many other neurological disorders, each with its unique set of symptoms and causes.
- The exact reasons why these diseases develop are still being researched, but factors like genetics, age, and lifestyle may play a role.
- There is currently no cure for any of these conditions, but there are treatments available to manage symptoms and improve quality of life.

A Glimmer of Hope:

Researchers worldwide are actively investigating these and other neurological disorders. As we gain a deeper understanding of the brain and these conditions, new treatment options and even preventative measures may emerge in the future.

The impact of brain injuries

The human brain is a remarkable organ, but it's also delicate. A traumatic brain injury (TBI) can disrupt its intricate functioning, leading to a range of physical, cognitive, and emotional challenges. However, the brain also possesses a powerful capacity for recovery, offering hope for those who have sustained a TBI.

The Scars of Trauma: Understanding TBI Effects

TBIs can occur from a blow to the head, a jolt to the body, or anything that disrupts normal brain function. The severity of the injury determines the extent of the impact, but some common effects include:

- **Physical:** Loss of consciousness, headaches, dizziness, sleep disturbances, and impaired balance or coordination.
- **Cognitive:** Difficulty concentrating, problems with memory and learning, confusion, and impaired judgment.
- **Emotional:** Anxiety, depression, irritability, personality changes, and difficulty managing emotions.
- **Communication:** Speech and language difficulties.

The Road to Recovery: Harnessing the Brain's Potential

The good news is that the brain has a remarkable ability to heal itself. This process, called neuroplasticity, involves the brain forming new connections and reorganizing itself to compensate for damaged areas. Here are some factors that can influence recovery:

- **Severity of the Injury:** The extent of damage plays a significant role. More severe TBIs may require longer and more intensive rehabilitation.

- **Timely Intervention:** Early diagnosis and intervention with rehabilitation programs can significantly improve outcomes.
- **Rehabilitation Strategies:** Physical, occupational, speech, and cognitive therapy can help individuals relearn skills and regain lost functions.
- **Individual Factors:** Age, overall health, and pre-injury cognitive reserve (brain health) can all influence the recovery process.

Living with TBI: Support and Hope

Living with a TBI can be challenging, but with support and a commitment to rehabilitation, individuals can lead fulfilling lives. Here are some key points to remember:

- **Support Systems:** Family, friends, and support groups can provide emotional encouragement and practical assistance.
- **Lifestyle Changes:** Healthy sleep habits, a balanced diet, and regular exercise can promote overall well-being and support brain recovery.
- **Self-Advocacy:** Learning about TBI and advocating for oneself can empower individuals to navigate the healthcare system and access necessary resources.

Remember:

- Recovery from a TBI is a journey, not a destination. It takes time, patience, and a dedicated effort.

- There is no one-size-fits-all approach to recovery. The rehabilitation plan will be tailored to the individual's specific needs and goals.
- With the right support and a commitment to recovery, individuals with TBI can regain function, improve their quality of life, and thrive.

Chapter 7
Fueling Your Brain Machine

The brain on a diet

The human brain is a power-hungry organ, and just like a high-performance car, it needs the right fuel to run at its best. Mounting evidence suggests a strong link between nutrition and brain health. Let's explore how what we eat can impact our cognitive function and the specific nutrients that play a crucial role:

The Gut-Brain Connection:

The gut microbiome, the community of trillions of microbes living in our intestines, plays a surprising role in brain health. These microbes influence the production of certain neurotransmitters, like serotonin, which impacts mood and learning. A healthy gut microbiome can promote better cognitive function, while an unhealthy gut can contribute to cognitive decline. Diet plays a significant role in shaping the gut microbiome composition.

Nutrient Powerhouse for the Brain:

Here are some key nutrients and their impact on cognitive function:

- **Omega-3 Fatty Acids:** Found in fatty fish, walnuts, and flaxseeds, omega-3s are essential for building and maintaining brain cell membranes. They may improve memory, learning, and protect against cognitive decline.
- **B Vitamins:** Vitamin B12, B6, and folate are crucial for neurotransmitter production and nerve function. Deficiencies can lead to fatigue, memory problems, and depression.
- **Antioxidants:** Found in fruits, vegetables, and whole grains, antioxidants help protect brain cells from damage caused by free radicals. This may contribute to improved memory and focus.
- **Choline:** Found in eggs, liver, and some vegetables, choline is a precursor to the neurotransmitter acetylcholine, which plays a vital role in memory, learning, and muscle control.
- **Flavanols:** Found in cocoa, green tea, and berries, flavanols may improve blood flow to the brain and enhance cognitive function, especially memory and learning.

Diet Patterns for Brain Health:

Several dietary patterns have been linked to improved cognitive function and a reduced risk of dementia. These include:

- **Mediterranean Diet:** Rich in fruits, vegetables, whole grains, healthy fats, and fish, this diet may benefit memory and cognitive function due to its anti-inflammatory and antioxidant properties.
- **DASH Diet:** Designed to lower blood pressure, the DASH diet (Dietary Approaches to Stop Hypertension) emphasizes fruits, vegetables, whole grains, and low-fat dairy products. It may also contribute to cognitive health.

Beyond Specific Nutrients:

It's important to remember that overall dietary patterns are more significant than focusing on single nutrients. Here are some additional points to consider:

- **Moderation is Key:** Limiting unhealthy fats, processed foods, and added sugars can significantly benefit brain health.
- **Hydration Matters:** Drinking plenty of water is crucial for optimal brain function. Dehydration can impair cognitive performance.
- **Variety is the Spice of Life:** Eating a diverse range of healthy foods ensures a wider range of nutrients for brain health.

By understanding the link between nutrition and brain health, we can make informed dietary choices to fuel our brains for optimal cognitive function and potentially reduce the risk of cognitive decline. Remember, a healthy brain starts on your plate!

Move it or lose it!

The saying "move it or lose it" isn't just about physical fitness; it applies to your brain health as well. Regular physical exercise offers a multitude of benefits for the body, and one of the most significant is its positive impact on the brain. Here's how getting your sweat on can boost your brainpower and promote neuroplasticity, the brain's ability to adapt and change.

Exercise: A Spark for the Brain

When you engage in physical activity, a cascade of positive changes occurs within your brain:

- **Increased Blood Flow:** Exercise gets your heart pumping, delivering a surge of oxygen and essential nutrients to the brain. This improved blood flow nourishes brain cells and promotes the growth of new blood vessels.
- **Neurotransmitter Boost:** Physical activity stimulates the production of neurotransmitters like dopamine, serotonin, and brain-derived neurotrophic factor (BDNF). These chemicals play a crucial role in learning, memory, mood regulation, and overall cognitive function.
- **Brain Cell Growth:** Regular exercise can actually lead to the growth of new brain cells, particularly in the hippocampus, which is essential for memory and learning.
- **Enhanced Neuroplasticity:** Exercise strengthens existing neural connections and

promotes the formation of new ones. This neuroplasticity allows the brain to adapt, learn new skills, and recover from damage.

The Benefits Beyond the Sweat:

The cognitive benefits of exercise are numerous:

- **Improved Memory and Learning:** Exercise can enhance your ability to learn new things, retain information, and recall memories more effectively.
- **Sharper Focus and Concentration:** Physical activity can improve your attention span, helping you focus better and filter out distractions.
- **Enhanced Problem-Solving Skills:** Exercise can stimulate cognitive flexibility, allowing you to approach problems creatively and find solutions more readily.
- **Reduced Risk of Cognitive Decline:** Regular exercise may help protect against age-related cognitive decline and neurodegenerative diseases like Alzheimer's.
- **Improved Mood and Reduced Stress:** Exercise is a natural mood booster, promoting the release of endorphins and reducing stress hormones. This can lead to a more positive outlook and better emotional well-being.

Getting Started with Exercise for Brainpower:

The good news is that you don't need to become a gym rat to reap the brain benefits of exercise. Even moderate physical activity can make a difference. Here are some tips:

- **Find an Activity You Enjoy:** The key is to choose activities you find fun and can stick with consistently. This could be anything from brisk walking, swimming, dancing, cycling, or team sports.
- **Aim for at Least 30 Minutes Most Days:** The Centers for Disease Control and Prevention (CDC) recommends at least 150 minutes of moderate-intensity aerobic activity or 75 minutes of vigorous-intensity aerobic activity per week. Even shorter bursts of activity, like taking the stairs or doing some jumping jacks during the day, can be beneficial.
- Include Strength Training: You must remember to incorporate strength training! Additionally, cognitive function can also benefit from the development of muscles. The goal should be to engage in workouts that focus on all the major muscle groups at least twice every week.

Move Your Body, Empower Your Brain

By incorporating regular physical activity into your routine, you're not just strengthening your body; you're giving your brain a powerful boost. Exercise promotes neuroplasticity, enhances cognitive function, and improves overall mental well-being. So, lace up your shoes, put on your favorite tunes, and get moving! Your brain will thank you for it.

Chapter 8
Keeping Your Brain Sharp

Lifelong learning

Our brains, like any muscle, need exercise to stay strong and healthy. While physical activity is crucial, mental stimulation plays an equally important role. Lifelong learning, the act of continuously engaging your mind with new information and experiences, offers a wealth of benefits for brain health and cognitive reserve.

The Importance of Mental Stimulation:

Our brains thrive on challenges. When we engage in mentally stimulating activities, we create new neural pathways, strengthen existing connections between brain cells, and stimulate the growth of new brain cells (neurogenesis) – all essential for optimal cognitive function. Here's how mental stimulation benefits the brain:

- **Enhanced Memory and Learning:** Learning new things keeps your memory sharp and improves your ability to learn and retain information.

- **Improved Focus and Concentration:** Regularly challenging your brain can enhance your ability to focus and concentrate, even on complex tasks.
- **Sharper Problem-Solving Skills:** Mental stimulation helps you approach problems from new angles and develop creative solutions.
- **Delayed Age-Related Cognitive Decline:** Studies suggest that lifelong learning can help delay the onset and progression of dementia and Alzheimer's disease.

Building Cognitive Reserve: A Brainpower Shield

Cognitive reserve refers to the brain's ability to adapt and compensate for changes or damage. It's like having a mental safety net. People with a higher cognitive reserve are better equipped to handle age-related decline and maintain cognitive function for longer. Lifelong learning is a key contributor to building a robust cognitive reserve:

- **Increased Brain Flexibility:** Mental stimulation promotes brain plasticity, allowing your brain to adapt to new situations and challenges.
- **Enhanced Neural Efficiency:** Regularly exercising your brain helps it work more efficiently, using fewer resources to achieve the same task.
- **Compensation for Damage:** A strong cognitive reserve allows the brain to compensate for

damage caused by aging or disease, minimizing the impact on cognitive function.

Lifelong Learning Doesn't Have to Be Formal:

The good news is that lifelong learning doesn't have to involve textbooks and classrooms. Here are some ways to keep your mind stimulated and build your cognitive reserve:

- **Learn a New Skill:** Take a class on anything that interests you, from painting to coding to a new language.
- **Read Regularly:** Reading exposes you to new ideas, expands your vocabulary, and keeps your mind engaged.
- **Play Brain Games:** Games that challenge your memory, logic, and problem-solving skills can be a fun way to exercise your brain.
- **Engage in Creative Activities:** Activities like painting, writing, or playing music tap into different parts of your brain and promote creativity.
- **Travel and Explore:** Experiencing new cultures, places, and people broadens your horizons and challenges your brain in new ways.

Brain-training games and activities

Brain-training games and puzzles have exploded in popularity, promising to enhance memory, focus, and cognitive function. But do they live up to the hype? Let's look into the potential benefits and limitations of these activities:

Potential Benefits:

- **Improved Processing Speed:** Some brain-training games that focus on reaction time and visual attention may lead to modest improvements in processing speed for specific tasks similar to those practiced in the game.
- **Enhanced Cognitive Skills:** Certain brain-training programs that target specific cognitive skills, like memory or problem-solving, might lead to improvements in those particular areas. However, the benefits may not transfer broadly to other cognitive skills.
- **Maintaining Cognitive Function:** Brain-training games can be a fun and engaging way to mentally stimulate older adults, potentially helping to maintain cognitive function and reduce the risk of age-related decline, although the evidence for this is not conclusive.

Limitations and Considerations:

- **Limited Transfer of Benefits:** The skills practiced in brain-training games may not translate to real-world situations. For example, improving your performance in a memory game might not necessarily translate to better recall of everyday tasks.
- **Focus on Specific Skills:** Brain-training games often target isolated cognitive skills, while real-world cognitive function relies on a complex interplay of various skills working together.
- **Overblown Claims:** Many brain-training programs make exaggerated claims about preventing dementia or boosting IQ. These claims are often not supported by robust scientific evidence.
- **Cost and Time Commitment:** Some brain-training programs require subscriptions or in-app purchases. The effectiveness of these programs can vary, and the time commitment required for potential benefits needs to be considered.

Beyond Brain-Training Games:

While brain-training games can be a fun addition to your mental fitness routine, they shouldn't be the sole focus for brain health. Here are some other strategies to consider:

- **Lifelong Learning:** Continuously challenge your mind by learning new skills, reading, or engaging in intellectually stimulating activities.
- **Physical Exercise:** Regular physical activity promotes blood flow to the brain, which can benefit cognitive function and overall brain health.
- **Healthy Diet:** Eating a balanced diet rich in fruits, vegetables, and whole grains provides essential nutrients that support brain health.
- **Quality Sleep:** Getting enough quality sleep is crucial for cognitive function and memory consolidation.
- **Social Interaction:** Engaging in social activities and maintaining strong social connections can stimulate the brain and promote cognitive well-being.

Here are some brain-training games that you can play without a device:

Memory Games:

- **Mental Math:** Challenge yourself with multiplication tables, addition or subtraction problems, or try calculating tips in your head while splitting a bill.

- **Kim's Game:** Place a variety of objects on a tray for a minute, then cover them. Try to recall and name all the objects after they are hidden. This can be done with household items or while playing a game of I Spy on a walk.
- **Rhyme Time:** Take turns thinking of words that rhyme with a chosen word. This is a fun activity to do with others and can be adapted to different categories (e.g., cities, fruits, animals).

Logic and Problem-Solving Games:

- **Sudoku on Paper:** Sudoku puzzles can be found in newspapers, magazines, or printed from websites.
- **Logic Puzzles:** Many logic puzzles can be found online and printed for offline use. These puzzles often involve solving riddles or mysteries using clues and deduction.
- **Mazes:** Mazes challenge you to find the path from start to finish. Look for them in puzzle books or magazines, or find printable mazes online.

Focus and Attention Games:

- **People Watching:** Find a public place and observe people's actions, clothing styles, or conversations. Try to remember details about the people you see after a set time.
- **Cloud Gazing:** Lie down and spend some time identifying shapes and formations in the clouds.

Let your imagination run wild and create stories based on the cloud shapes.
- **Counting Challenges:** Set a timer for a minute and see how many objects you can count in your environment (e.g., trees in a park, red cars on the street).

Bonus: Creative Activities

- **Storytelling:** Take turns with someone adding sentences to a story, building a narrative together.
- **Drawing Games:** Play Pictionary or similar games where you describe a word or phrase for someone else to draw, or take turns adding details to a collaborative drawing.
- **Crosswords:** Look for crossword puzzles in newspapers or magazines, or print them from websites.

These are just a few ideas to get you started. There are many other brain-training activities that can be done without a device.

Sleep for success

Sleep isn't just a period of inactivity; it's a vital process crucial for our physical and mental well-being. During sleep, our brains are incredibly active, consolidating memories, processing information, and flushing out toxins. Let's look into the crucial role sleep plays in memory consolidation and overall brain function:

Memory Consolidation: Locking in the Lessons of the Day

While we're awake, our brains are bombarded with information. Sleep allows us to process and consolidate these experiences into memories. This consolidation process happens in several stages:

- **Short-Term Storage:** New information is temporarily stored in the hippocampus, a brain region crucial for memory formation.
- **Replay and Reactivation:** During sleep, especially during deep sleep stages, the brain replays and reactivates these short-term memories.
- **Strengthening Connections:** These replays strengthen the connections between neurons, solidifying the information and transitioning it into long-term memory storage in the cortex.

Sleep Deprivation: Disrupting the Memory Machine

When we don't get enough sleep, this memory consolidation process is disrupted. Here's how sleep deprivation can negatively impact memory:

- **Difficulty Forming Memories:** The brain struggles to encode new information into short-term memory, making it harder to form new memories in the first place.
- **Fragile Memories:** Memories formed during sleep deprivation are weaker and more likely to be forgotten.
- **Impaired Recall:** The ability to retrieve and recall stored memories can be significantly hindered by a lack of sleep.

Beyond Memory: The Widespread Benefits of Sleep

Sleep's benefits extend far beyond memory consolidation. Here are some other ways sleep impacts brain function:

- **Learning and Creativity:** Sleep facilitates the brain's ability to learn new skills and information. It also plays a role in creative problem-solving and thinking outside the box.
- **Emotional Regulation:** Sleep deprivation can worsen mood swings and make it harder to manage stress and emotions. Adequate sleep promotes emotional well-being and resilience.
- **Focus and Concentration:** A well-rested brain is better equipped to focus, concentrate, and pay attention. Sleep deprivation can lead to

decreased alertness, making it harder to concentrate on tasks.
- **Decision-Making:** Sleep deprivation can impair our ability to make sound decisions and judgments. Adequate sleep allows for clearer thinking and better decision-making skills.

Investing in Sleep for Optimal Brain Function

Making sleep a priority is an investment in your overall brain health and cognitive function. Here are some tips for promoting better sleep:

- **Set up a Regular Sleep Schedule:** Try to retire and get up at the same period every day including weekends. This assists in regulating your body's natural sleep-wake cycle.
- **Develop a Relaxing Pre-sleep Routine:** Do quiet things before going to bed, such as reading, taking a hot bath or practicing relaxation techniques.
- **Optimize Your Sleep Environment:** Ensure your bedroom is dark, quiet, cool, and clutter-free to promote better sleep quality.
- **Limit Screen Time Before Bed:** The blue light emitted from electronic devices can disrupt sleep patterns. Make sure you don't get glued to any screen at least an hour before going to bed.
- **Regular Exercise:** Regular physical activity can improve sleep quality, but avoid strenuous exercise too close to bedtime.

Unbreakable power of the brain

Chapter 9
Taming Stress and Embracing Mindfulness

The stress monster and the brain

Chronic stress can feel like a relentless monster, draining our energy and impacting our mood. But beyond the emotional toll, chronic stress can also wreak havoc on our brains, affecting memory, focus, and even shrinking brain volume. Let's delve into the ways chronic stress negatively impacts brain function:

Stress Hormones:

When we face a stressful situation, our body releases a surge of hormones like cortisol. This prepares us to deal with the threat, sharpening our focus and alertness. However, chronic stress keeps these hormones elevated for extended periods, disrupting the delicate balance in the brain.

- **Cortisol and Hippocampal Shrinkage:** Chronically high cortisol levels can shrink the hippocampus, a brain region crucial for memory formation and learning. This can lead to

difficulty forming new memories, problems with recall, and impaired learning.
- **Reduced Neurogenesis:** Stress can hinder the brain's ability to create new neurons, a process called neurogenesis. This is particularly important for the hippocampus and can contribute to cognitive decline.

Brain Fog and Impaired Thinking:

Chronic stress can create a persistent state of "brain fog," making it difficult to concentrate, focus, and think clearly. Here's how:

- **Disrupted Prefrontal Cortex Function:** The prefrontal cortex is responsible for executive functions like planning, decision-making, and problem-solving. Chronic stress can impair its function, leading to difficulties with these tasks.
- **Reduced Cognitive Flexibility:** Stress can make it harder to adapt to new situations and think creatively. The brain gets stuck in a "fight-or-flight" mode, hindering its ability to process information and respond flexibly.

The Domino Effect:

Chronic stress can exacerbate or even trigger mental health problems like anxiety and depression. These conditions further disrupt brain function, creating a vicious cycle.

- **Stress and Anxiety:** Chronic stress can lead to anxiety, which can manifest as racing thoughts, difficulty concentrating, and sleep problems.
- **Stress and Depression:** Stress can be a major contributor to depression, which can lead to feelings of hopelessness, low motivation, and difficulty experiencing pleasure. These symptoms can further impair cognitive function.

Combating the Stress Monster: Strategies for Brain Protection

While chronic stress can be damaging, there's good news: we can learn to manage stress and protect our brains. Here are some strategies:

- **Stress Management Techniques:** Practices like meditation, yoga, and deep breathing can help reduce stress hormones and promote relaxation.
- **Physical Activity:** Regular exercise is a powerful stress reliever and can also boost cognitive function.
- **Healthy Diet:** Eating a balanced diet rich in fruits, vegetables, and whole grains provides the brain with the nutrients it needs to function optimally.
- **Quality Sleep:** Adequate sleep allows the brain to repair itself and recover from the effects of stress.
- **Social Support:** Strong social connections provide emotional support and can buffer the negative effects of stress.

Relaxation techniques for a calmer you

Life can be a whirlwind of deadlines, demands, and obligations. In the midst of it all, feeling stressed, overwhelmed, and anxious is perfectly normal. But chronic stress can take a toll on our physical and mental well-being. Thankfully, there are a range of relaxation techniques that can help us cultivate inner peace, manage stress, and promote a calmer state of mind. Let's explore some powerful tools for your relaxation toolbox:

Mindfulness: Anchoring Yourself in the Present Moment

Mindfulness is the practice of paying attention to the present moment without judgment. It's about becoming aware of your thoughts, feelings, and bodily sensations without getting caught up in them. Here are some ways to cultivate mindfulness:

- **Mindful Breathing:** Focus on your breath, feeling the rise and fall of your chest or abdomen with each inhalation and exhalation. This simple practice can help anchor you in the present moment and promote relaxation.
- **Mindful Movement:** Activities like yoga or tai chi combine physical movement with mindfulness. By focusing on your body and its sensations as you move, you can quiet your mind and reduce stress.

- **Mindful Eating:** Slow down and savor your food, paying attention to the taste, texture, and smell. This not only promotes mindful eating habits but can also be a calming and grounding experience.

Meditation: Training Your Mind for Calmness

Meditation is a practice that involves focusing your attention and quieting your mind. There are many different meditation techniques, but some common ones include:

- **Focused Attention Meditation:** Focus your attention on an object, mantra (a repeated word or phrase), or your breath. When your mind wanders, gently bring your attention back to your chosen focus point.
- **Loving-Kindness Meditation:** Cultivate feelings of kindness and compassion towards yourself and others. This practice can promote positive emotions and reduce stress.
- **Guided Meditation:** Listen to guided meditations that lead you through a visualization or relaxation exercise. These can be a great way for beginners to get started with meditation.

Beyond Mindfulness and Meditation: Relaxation Techniques for Everyone

While mindfulness and meditation are powerful tools, there are many other relaxation techniques you can explore:

- **Progressive Muscle Relaxation:** Tense and relax different muscle groups in your body, starting with your toes and working your way up. This can help release physical tension and promote relaxation.
- **Deep Breathing Exercises:** Practice slow, diaphragmatic breathing. Inhale through your nose for a count of four, hold for a count of seven, and exhale slowly through your mouth for a count of eight.
- **Visualization:** Imagine yourself in a peaceful and calming setting. This can help reduce stress and promote relaxation.
- **Spending Time in Nature:** Immersing yourself in nature has been shown to reduce stress and improve mood. Take a walk in the park, sit by a stream, or simply gaze at the clouds.
- **Engaging in Hobbies:** Activities you enjoy can take your mind off your worries and promote relaxation. Whether it's reading, painting, listening to music, or spending time with loved ones, find activities that bring you joy and peace.

Finding What Works for You:

The key to relaxation is finding techniques that resonate with you. Experiment with different methods and see what helps you feel calmer and more centered. Remember, relaxation is a skill that takes practice. Be patient with yourself and incorporate these techniques into your daily routine for a more peaceful and stress-free you.

Chapter 10
The Cutting Edge of Brain Research

Exploring the frontiers

Neuroscience is a field brimming with exciting advancements. Scientists are constantly pushing the boundaries of our understanding of the brain, developing groundbreaking technologies and potential treatments for neurological disorders. Let's delve into some of these frontiers:

Brain-Computer Interfaces (BCIs): Bridging the Mind-Machine Gap

BCIs are devices that directly translate brain activity into commands that can control external devices. Imagine controlling a prosthetic limb, a wheelchair, or even a computer just by thinking about it! Here's a glimpse into the world of BCIs:

- **Non-Invasive BCIs:** These BCIs use techniques like electroencephalography (EEG) to read brain signals from the scalp. While they may not be as powerful as invasive BCIs, they offer more practicality for everyday use.
- **Invasive BCIs:** These BCIs involve implanting electrodes directly into the brain, allowing for a more precise and powerful signal. However, they are more complex and carry a higher surgical risk.

The Potential Applications of BCIs are Vast:

- **Restoring Movement and Communication:** BCIs offer immense hope for individuals with paralysis, spinal cord injuries, or ALS (amyotrophic lateral sclerosis) by allowing them to control prosthetic limbs or communication devices.
- **Assistive Technologies:** BCIs could be used to control wheelchairs, smart homes, or other assistive technologies through thought alone.
- **Gaming and Entertainment:** BCIs could revolutionize the gaming industry, allowing for a more immersive and interactive experience.

Ethical Considerations of BCIs:

The potential of BCIs raises important ethical questions. Issues like privacy, security, and the potential for misuse of brain data need careful consideration.

Hope on the Horizon: Potential Treatments for Neurological Disorders

Brain research is also leading to breakthroughs in treatments for various neurological disorders:

- **Alzheimer's Disease:** Researchers are exploring new drugs and therapies targeting the underlying causes of Alzheimer's, such as amyloid plaque buildup and tau protein tangles.
- **Parkinson's Disease:** Gene therapy and deep brain stimulation are being investigated as potential treatments to alleviate the symptoms of Parkinson's.
- **Depression:** New neuromodulation techniques, like transcranial magnetic stimulation (TMS), offer promise for treating treatment-resistant depression.

These advancements are just the tip of the iceberg. Brain research is a rapidly evolving field, and the future holds even more exciting possibilities. With continued research and development, we can hope to unlock the full potential of the brain and improve the lives of millions suffering from neurological disorders.

Ethical considerations

The potential of brain enhancement technologies like BCIs and nootropics (cognitive enhancement drugs) is undeniable. However, alongside the promise lies a complex web of ethical considerations that demand careful attention:

- **Equity and Access:** Brain enhancement technologies may be expensive and inaccessible to large portions of the population. This could exacerbate social inequalities and create an "enhanced" elite.
- **Informed Consent:** Brain enhancement can have unforeseen consequences. Ensuring individuals fully understand the potential risks and benefits before undergoing any procedures or taking medications is crucial.
- **Cognitive Liberty:** Does enhancing your brain become a societal pressure or expectation? Should individuals have the freedom to choose not to enhance their brains?
- **Blurring the Lines of Natural and Artificial:** If brain-computer interfaces become commonplace, how will we define what it means to be human? Where do we draw the line between natural cognitive function and artificial enhancement?
- **Weaponization of Brain Tech:** The potential for misuse of brain-computer interfaces for military or malicious purposes needs careful consideration and safeguards.

Conclusion

Our brains are not static organs; they are remarkably plastic and adaptable throughout life. Here's a quick recap of the key takeaways about this incredible potential:

- **Neuroplasticity:** The brain's ability to change and reorganize itself in response to experiences, learning, and challenges.
- **Benefits of Exercise:** Physical activity promotes neurogenesis (growth of new brain cells), strengthens neural connections, and improves cognitive function.
- **Lifelong Learning:** Continuously stimulating your mind with new activities keeps your brain sharp, builds cognitive reserve, and may help delay age-related decline.
- **Importance of Sleep:** Adequate sleep is crucial for memory consolidation, information processing, and overall brain function.
- **Managing Stress:** Chronic stress can negatively impact memory, focus, and even shrink brain volume. Learning stress-management techniques is vital for brain health.

By understanding the brain's plasticity and incorporating practices that promote its well-being, we can unlock its full potential and empower ourselves to learn, grow, and thrive throughout life.

The human brain is a universe contained within our skulls. It is a complex and awe-inspiring organ, capable of breathtaking feats of creativity, reason, and emotion. As we unravel its mysteries, let's remember the words of Santiago Ramón y Cajal, the father of modern neuroscience: "Every man is, to some extent, the architect of his own brain." Through our choices, habits, and experiences, we have the power to shape and optimize this incredible organ. So, embark on your brain optimization journey, unlock its potential, and together, let's rewrite the narrative of what it means to be human.

I Have a Request

We Value Your Feedback!

We hope you're enjoying your journey through "Unbreakable power of the brain" and learning amazing things about the incredible human brain!

Your honest feedback is incredibly valuable to us. It helps us understand what readers like you find helpful and inspiring, and it allows others to make informed decisions about whether this book is the right book for them.

Would you be willing to share your thoughts on Amazon?
Here's how you can leave a review:
1. Go to your Amazon account and navigate to "Your Orders."
2. Find your purchase of "Unbreakable power of the brain" and click on it.
3. Scroll down to the "Product Reviews" section and click on "Write a review."
4. Share your honest thoughts about the book - what you liked, what you found helpful, or anything else you'd like to mention.

Thank you for taking the time to consider sharing your feedback. We appreciate your support!

Sincerely,
Charles Porras

www.ingramcontent.com/pod-product-compliance
Lightning Source LLC
Chambersburg PA
CBHW071215240526
45470CB00018B/1868